The Complete Guide to Holistic Wellness

Achieving Balance in Mind, Body, and Spirit

By Maya Harmony

The Complete Guide to Holistic Wellness by Maya Harmony

The Complete Guide to Holistic Wellness by Maya Harmony

Copyright

Copyright © 2024 by Maya Harmony

Disclaimer

The information provided in this book is for educational and informational purposes only and is not intended as a substitute for professional medical advice, diagnosis, or treatment. Always seek the advice of your physician or other qualified health care provider with any questions you may have regarding a medical condition or treatment and before undertaking a new health care regimen. The author and publisher of this book are not responsible for any adverse effects or consequences resulting from the use of the information contained herein. Each individual's health and wellness journey is unique, and readers are encouraged to consult with appropriate health professionals to determine what may be best for their specific needs.

The Complete Guide to Holistic Wellness by Maya Harmony

4

The Complete Guide to Holistic Wellness by Maya Harmony

About the Author

Dr. Maya Harmony is a passionate advocate for holistic wellness, dedicated to helping others achieve balance and vitality in mind, body, and spirit. With a background in holistic medicine, naturopathy, integrative health, wellness coaching, Dr. Harmony combines her expertise with a deep commitment to empowering individuals to reclaim their health and well-being naturally. Through her work as a holistic wellness practitioner, she has touched the lives of countless individuals, guiding them on their journey to radiant wellness. Driven by a profound belief in the interconnectedness of all things, Dr. Harmony's mission is to inspire and uplift others as they embark on their own paths to holistic living.

The Complete Guide to Holistic Wellness by Maya Harmony

INTRODUCTION

In a world teeming with hustle and bustle, where time races forward relentlessly and demands seem never-ending, there exists a quiet whisper, a gentle reminder of a different path—the path of holistic wellness. It's a journey that beckons us to pause, to listen to the whispers of our souls, and to embark on a quest for balance, harmony, and vitality in mind, body, and spirit.

Picture yourself standing at the edge of a lush forest, the air thick with the scent of pine and earth, the sunlight filtering through the canopy above, casting dappled shadows on the forest floor. As you step onto the winding path before you, you can feel the earth beneath your feet, grounding you, connecting you to the pulse of life that thrums through every living thing.

Holistic wellness is not merely the absence of illness; it is a state of vibrant health and vitality that encompasses every aspect of our being. It is the recognition that we are not merely physical bodies, but intricate being's woven from the threads of our thoughts, emotions, beliefs, and experiences. To truly thrive, we must nurture each of these threads, weaving them together into a tapestry of wholeness and well-being.

As you journey deeper into the forest of holistic wellness, you will encounter ancient wisdom passed down through the ages—wisdom that speaks to the interconnectedness of all things, the delicate dance of energy that flows through the universe, binding us all together in a web of existence.

At its core, holistic wellness is about honoring the innate wisdom of the body, mind, and spirit, and cultivating practices that support their natural balance and harmony. It is about nourishing ourselves with whole foods that nourish not only our bodies but also our souls. It is about moving our bodies with joy and intention, honoring the miraculous vessel that carries us through life's journey. It is about finding moments of stillness and silence amidst the chaos of daily life, allowing us to reconnect with our innermost selves and the wisdom that resides within.

But holistic wellness is not a destination; it is a journey—a journey of self-discovery, self-care, and self-compassion. It is a journey that invites us to embrace the fullness of our humanity—the light and the shadow, the joy and the sorrow, the triumphs and the challenges—and to find beauty and meaning in every moment.

As you continue along the path of holistic wellness, know that you are not alone. You are part of a vast and interconnected web of beings, all walking this journey together. And though the path may be winding and at times challenging, know that every step you take brings you closer to the radiant vitality and profound sense of well-being that awaits you at the journey's end. **So let's get started**

Chapter 1

Deep within the very center of our being lies a profound truth: the mind and body are not separate entities but interconnected parts of our existence, forever intertwined in a dance of mutual influence and feedback. In this chapter, we embark on a journey of exploration, delving into the intricate web of connections that bind our thoughts, emotions, and physical well-being.

The Mind-Body Continuum: Bridging the Gap Between Thoughts and Health

Imagine waking up one morning feeling a bit under the weather. Maybe you're feeling a little stressed about an upcoming deadline at work, or perhaps you had an argument with a loved one the night before. As you go about your day, you notice that your shoulders feel tense, your stomach churns uneasily, and your head throbs with a dull ache. It's as ifyour body is sending you a message.

Welcome to the world of the mind-body continuum, where the lines between thoughts and physical health blur. In this intricate balance of interconnectedness, every thought, feeling, and sensation we experience has the potential to influence our physical well-being, shaping the landscape of our health in ways both subtle and profound.

At the heart of the mind-body continuum lies the recognition that our mental and emotional states are not isolated phenomena but powerful forces that sculpt the terrain of our physical health. Take stress, for example. When we encounter a perceived threat—a looming deadline, a conflict with a colleague—our body springs into action, initiating the stress response. Adrenaline floods our bloodstream, our heart races, and our muscles tense, preparing us to confront the perceived danger head-on.

In the short term, this stress response is adaptive, helping us to mobilize our resources and navigate the challenges of everyday life. But when stress becomes chronic—a constant companion in our modern, fast-paced world—it can exact a heavy toll on our health. Research has linked chronic stress to a host of health problems, including cardiovascular disease, immune dysfunction, and gastrointestinal disorders, underscoring the profound impact of our mental and emotional states on our physical well-being.

But the mind-body continuum is not a one-way street; it is a dynamic, bidirectional highway of influence, where the body's state can also shape our thoughts and emotions. Consider the experience of chronic pain, for instance. For someone living with persistent physical discomfort, the relentless drumbeat of pain can color every aspect of their existence, casting a shadow over even the brightest moments of joy. In this way, the body's state can shape the landscape of our inner world, influencing our thoughts, emotions, and perceptions in profound ways.

But amidst the complexities of the mind-body continuum lies a glimmer of hope—a recognition of the transformative power we hold within ourselves. Through practices such as mindfulness meditation, yoga, and deep breathing, we can learn to cultivate greater awareness of the mind-body connection, attuning to the subtle signals of our inner landscape and fostering a deeper sense of harmony and balance within ourselves.

As we journey deeper into the heart of the mind-body continuum, may we come to recognize the profound interconnectedness of our existence and harness the power of this dynamic relationship to cultivate vibrant health, resilience, and well-being in every aspect of our lives.

Stress and the Body: Navigating the Tumultuous Waters of Modern Life

Picture this: You're sitting in traffic, the minutes ticking by as you inch forward at a snail's pace. Your mind races with thoughts of all the tasks awaiting you at work, the mounting deadlines, the endless to-do lists. Your heart pounds in your chest, your muscles tense with frustration, and a wave of exhaustion washes over you. Welcome to the world of stress—a ubiquitous companion in our modern, fast-paced lives.

Stress is a natural response to perceived threats, a primal survival mechanism that has helped humans navigate the challenges of our evolutionary past. When faced with a predator or a rival tribe, our ancestors relied on the stress response to mobilize their resources, enabling them to fight or flee with speed and agility.

But in today's world, the threats we face are often more subtle and insidious—a demanding boss, a looming deadline, financial worries—and yet, our bodies respond with the same primal intensity, triggering the cascade of physiological changes known as the stress response.

At the heart of the stress response lies the activation of the sympathetic nervous system, the body's rapid-response system for dealing with emergencies. When we perceive a threat, whether real or imagined, the sympathetic nervous system springs into action, releasing a surge of stress hormones such as adrenaline and cortisol into the bloodstream.

These hormones have far-reaching effects on the body, priming us for action by increasing heart rate, blood pressure, and respiration, and diverting energy away from non-essential functions such as digestion and immunity. This physiological surge is what gives us the burst of energy and focus we need to tackle the perceived threat head-on—the classic "fight or flight" response.

The Ripple Effect of Stress

But the impact of stress doesn't end with our physical health—it extends its tendrils into every corner of our lives, shaping our thoughts, emotions, and relationships in profound ways. Consider the experience of chronic stress on our mental and emotional well-being. As the pressures of life mount and the demands of work, family, and personal obligations pile up, it's all too easy to feel overwhelmed, anxious, and emotionally drained.

Chronic stress can take a toll on our mental health, contributing to feelings of anxiety, depression, and burnout. It can erode our sense of self-worth and confidence, leaving us feeling powerless and defeated in the face of life's challenges. It can also strain our relationships, as the tension and irritability that often accompany chronic stress spill over into our interactions with loved ones, leading to conflict and disconnection.

Breaking the Cycle

But amidst the storm clouds of stress, there exists a glimmer of hope—a recognition of our innate capacity for resilience and self-care. By cultivating practices such as mindfulness meditation, yoga, and deep breathing, we can learn to navigate the tumultuous waters of stress with greater ease and grace, fostering a sense of calm and equilibrium amidst the chaos.

Mindfulness meditation, in particular, has emerged as a powerful tool for managing stress and promoting emotional well-being. By bringing our attention to the present moment, without judgment or attachment, we can learn to observe our thoughts and emotions with greater clarity and compassion, cultivating a sense of inner peace and acceptance that transcends the turmoil of daily life.

Similarly, practices such as yoga and deep breathing can help to soothe the body's stress response, promoting relaxation and reducing the physical symptoms of stress such as muscle tension and elevated heart rate. By incorporating these practices into our daily routine, we can create a sanctuary of calm amidst the chaos of modern life, nurturing our well-being and fostering a sense of balance and harmony within ourselves.

The Power of Thoughts and Beliefs

Imagine your mind as a vast garden, teeming with seeds of thought and belief. With each passing moment, you sow these seeds into the fertile soil of your consciousness, unaware of the profound impact they may one day yield. Yet, beneath the surface, these seeds take root, sending forth forces of influence that shape the landscape of your reality.

Our thoughts and beliefs possess an extraordinary power—a power to shape our perceptions, influence our emotions, and ultimately, mold the fabric of our lived experience. Like master sculptors, we wield this power with every thought we entertain, every belief we hold dear, crafting the contours of our inner and outer worlds with exquisite precision.

The Science Behind the Magic

But what is it about thoughts and beliefs that makes them so potent? To understand their power, we must journey into the realm of neuroscience and psychology, where cutting-edge research illuminates the intricate workings of the human mind.

Studies in the field of psychoneuroimmunology have revealed the profound ways in which our thoughts and beliefs impact our physical health. For example, researchers have found that individuals who maintain a positive outlook tend to exhibit stronger immune function, faster recovery times from illness, and even greater longevity compared to their pessimistic counterparts. Conversely, those who harbor negative thought patterns and limiting beliefs may find themselves more susceptible to illness, experiencing higher levels of stress, inflammation, and disease.

The Power of Positive Thinking

Consider the simple act of cultivating a positive mindset. When we approach life with optimism and hope, we send a clear signal to our brains and bodies that all is well in our world. In response, our brains release a cascade of feel-good neurotransmitters, such as dopamine and serotonin, which uplift our mood and bolster our resilience in the face of adversity.

Moreover, positive thinking can have a ripple effect on our relationships, influencing how we perceive and interact with others. When we approach our interactions with kindness, empathy, and compassion, we create a positive feedback loop that fosters deeper connections and greater mutual understanding.

The Influence of Beliefs

Our beliefs, too, exert a profound influence on our reality. Whether conscious or subconscious, our beliefs act as filters through which we interpret the world around us, shaping our perceptions and coloring our experiences. For example, someone who holds a belief in their own unworthiness may perceive every setback as further evidence of their inadequacy, reinforcing a cycle of self-doubt and limitation.

Conversely, someone who holds a belief in their inherent worth and potential may approach challenges with resilience and determination, viewing each obstacle as an opportunity for growth and learning.

Harnessing the Power Within

In recognizing the immense power of our thoughts and beliefs, we are invited to become conscious creators of our reality. By cultivating mindfulness and self-awareness, we can begin to observe the patterns of thought and belief that shape our lives, discerning which serve our highest good and which no longer serve us. Through practices such as affirmation, visualization, and cognitive reframing, we can rewire our brains for positivity and possibility, paving the way for a life of greater joy, fulfillment, and well-being.
Emotions and the Body: The Dance of Inner Experience

Imagine a moment of pure joy—the exhilaration of laughter bubbling up from deep within, the warmth of connection enveloping you like a gentle embrace. In that moment, every cell in your body vibrates with life, infused with the radiant energy of your emotions. This is the power of emotions—the potent force that shapes our inner landscape and reverberates throughout our physical being.

The Language of Emotions

Emotions are the language of the soul, the vibrant hues that paint the canvas of our inner experience. From the fiery intensity of anger to the soft whisper of contentment, each emotion carries with it a unique energy signature that colors our perceptions and shapes our reality.

But emotions are not merely fleeting sensations; they are embodied experiences, woven into the very fabric of our being. Consider the sensation of fear—the rapid heartbeat, the shallow breath, the clammy palms—all visceral responses that arise in response to perceived threats, preparing the body to react with lightning speed.

The Physiology of Emotions

Behind every emotion lies a complex interplay of neurochemicals, hormones, and neural pathways, orchestrating a symphony of physiological responses throughout the body. When we experience joy, for example, the brain releases a flood of feel-good neurotransmitters such as dopamine and endorphins, eliciting feelings of pleasure and euphoria.

Conversely, emotions such as fear or anger trigger the activation of the sympathetic nervous system, initiating the body's fight-or-flight response. Adrenaline surges through the bloodstream, heart rate accelerates, and muscles tense in preparation for action—all adaptive responses designed to ensure our survival in the face of danger.

The Impact on Health

The profound interconnection between emotions and the body has far-reaching implications for our health and well-being. Chronic stress, for example, can dysregulate the body's stress response system, leading to a cascade of physiological imbalances that increase the risk of chronic diseases such as hypertension, diabetes, and depression.

Likewise, unexpressed or suppressed emotions can manifest as physical symptoms, manifesting as tension headaches, digestive disturbances, or muscle pain. By acknowledging and honoring our emotions, we can release the energetic blockages that impede the body's natural healing processes, restoring balance and vitality to mind, body, and spirit.

Cultivating Emotional Resilience

In the face of life's inevitable ups and downs, cultivating emotional resilience becomes essential. This entails developing the capacity to navigate the full spectrum of human emotions with grace and compassion, embracing each experience as an opportunity for growth and self-discovery.

Practices such as mindfulness meditation, journaling, and expressive arts can help us cultivate emotional awareness and regulation, enabling us to respond to life's challenges with greater equanimity and presence. By nurturing a deeper connection with our emotions and honoring the wisdom they hold, we can embark on a journey of healing and transformation that encompasses every aspect of our being.

Cultivating Mind-Body Awareness

Imagine sitting in a quiet room, the gentle rhythm of your breath serving as a steady anchor amidst the swirl of thoughts and sensations that dance through your mind. This is the practice of cultivating mind-body awareness—a journey of self-discovery and self-understanding that invites us to deepen our connection with the inner landscape of our bodies and minds.

At its core, mind-body awareness is about tuning into the subtle signals of the body and mind, learning to listen to the intuition and wisdom that reside within. It is about becoming attuned to the ebb and flow of sensations, emotions, and thoughts that course through our being, without judgment or attachment.

One powerful tool for cultivating mind-body awareness is mindfulness meditation. In mindfulness meditation, we bring our full attention to the present moment, anchoring our awareness in the sensations of the breath as it flows in and out of the body. With each breath, we become more deeply attuned to the sensations that arise within us—the rise and fall of the chest, the expansion and contraction of the belly, the subtle movements of energy that ripple through our being.

As we practice mindfulness meditation, we may notice that our minds are quick to wander, drifting into memories of the past or worries about the future. And that's okay. In mindfulness, we gently acknowledge these thoughts and gently guide our attention back to the present moment, returning again and again to the breath as our anchor.

Another powerful practice for cultivating mind-body awareness is body scanning. In body scanning, we systematically bring our attention to each part of the body, starting from the crown of the head and moving down to the tips of the toes. With each scan, we notice any sensations that arise—a twinge of tension in the shoulders, a flutter of warmth in the belly, a tingling sensation in the hands—and simply observe them without judgment or resistance.

Through practices like mindfulness meditation and body scanning, we begin to cultivate a deeper sense of connection with ourselves and the world around us. We become more attuned to the signals of our bodies, more aware of the thoughts and emotions that shape our experience, and more grounded in the present moment.

In our busy, fast-paced world, cultivating mind-body awareness is more important than ever. By taking the time to tune into the wisdom of our bodies and minds, we can navigate life's challenges with greater clarity, resilience, and grace. And as we deepen our connection with ourselves, we open the door to a world of possibility, where healing, growth, and transformation become not just aspirations, but lived realities.

Chapter 2

At the heart of holistic wellness lies the recognition that food is more than mere sustenance—it is medicine, energy, and connection. Each bite we take is an opportunity to nourish ourselves on a profound level, providing our bodies with the essential nutrients they need to thrive and flourish.

Let us begin by delving into the concept of nutrition, the science of how our bodies utilize the food we eat to fuel cellular function, support growth and repair, and maintain overall health. From the macronutrients—carbohydrates, proteins, and fats—that provide us with energy, to the micronutrients—vitamins, minerals, and phytonutrients—that play vital roles in countless biochemical processes, every nutrient has its part to play in the symphony of health.

But nutrition is not merely about counting calories or grams of fat; it is about nourishing ourselves on a deeper level, honoring the innate wisdom of our bodies and the unique needs of our individual constitutions. It is about listening to the whispers of hunger and satiety, tuning in to the signals our bodies send us to guide us toward foods that truly nourish and sustain us.

But nourishment extends beyond the physical realm; it encompasses the emotional and spiritual dimensions of our relationship with food as well. Let us explore the rituals and traditions that surround food in cultures around the world, from the communal gatherings that celebrate the harvest to the intimate moments shared over a home-cooked meal with loved ones.

In a world where diets and conflicting nutrition advice abound, let us reclaim our power to nourish ourselves in a way that honors our bodies and our souls. Let us approach food with mindfulness and intention, savoring each bite as a gift from the earth and a reflection of the interconnected web of life of which we are all a part.

Mindful eating invites us to bring a heightened awareness and presence to our meals, allowing us to fully engage with the sensory experience of eating and to cultivate a deeper connection to our bodies' hunger and satiety cues.

Intuitive nutrition encourages us to trust our bodies' innate wisdom and to honor our cravings and preferences without judgment or restriction. It empowers us to break free from the cycle of dieting and to embrace a more flexible and sustainable approach to nourishment that is rooted in self-compassion and self-care.

As we navigate the sea of dietary recommendations and nutritional guidelines, let us remember that there is no one-size-fits-all approach to nourishment. Each of us is unique, with our own individual needs, preferences, and tolerances. What works for one person may not work for another, and it is essential to honor and respect our bodies' wisdom as we explore what nourishment means for us.

In our modern world, where convenience often takes precedence over quality and quantity over substance, let us strive to reconnect with the wisdom of our ancestors, who lived in harmony with the rhythms of nature and honored the sacredness of food as both sustenance and medicine. Let us rediscover the joy of cooking and sharing meals with loved ones, and let us savor each bite as a celebration of life and vitality.

In this journey of nourishing the body, let us also explore the impact of our food choices on the health of the planet. As stewards of the earth, we have a responsibility to consider the environmental consequences of our dietary habits and to strive for sustainability and ethical consumption.

By choosing locally grown, seasonal produce and supporting regenerative agriculture practices, we can minimize our carbon footprint and help protect the delicate balance of ecosystems around the globe. Likewise, by reducing our consumption of animal products and opting for plant-based alternatives, we can mitigate the environmental impact of animal agriculture and promote the well-being of both animals and the planet.

In addition to its environmental benefits, a plant-based diet has been shown to offer numerous health advantages, including lower risk of chronic diseases such as heart disease, diabetes, and certain types of cancer. By incorporating more fruits, vegetables, whole grains, and legumes into our diets, we can boost our intake of essential nutrients and phytonutrients while reducing our intake of saturated fat, cholesterol, and processed foods.

But nourishment is not just about what we eat; it is also about how we relate to food and our bodies. In a culture that often equates thinness with health and moral virtue, it is essential to challenge harmful diet culture messages and embrace a more inclusive and compassionate approach to health and wellness. Let us celebrate our bodies in all their diverse shapes and sizes and cultivate a sense of gratitude for the incredible things they do for us each and every day.

As we journey onward in our quest for holistic wellness, let us remember that nourishing the body is a lifelong practice—an ever-unfolding journey of discovery, exploration, and growth. By approaching food with mindfulness, intention, and reverence, we can harness its transformative power to heal, energize, and inspire us on our path to radiant health and vitality.

Chapter 3

Physical activity is not just about breaking a sweat or building muscles; it is about honoring the inherent need of the body to move, to stretch, to breathe deeply, and to thrive.

Our bodies are marvels of engineering, designed for movement and activity. From the graceful arc of a dancer's leap to the powerful stride of a runner, our bodies are capable of an astonishing array of movements, each one a testament to the incredible potential that resides within us.

Physical activity is more than just a means to an end; it is a fundamental aspect of holistic wellness that nourishes not only our physical bodies but also our minds and spirits. When we move our bodies, we awaken dormant energies, release tension, and invigorate our senses. We feel alive, vibrant, and fully present in the moment.

But physical activity is not just about what happens during the workout; it is about the ripple effects that extend far beyond the confines of the gym or the yoga mat. Regular exercise has been shown to have a myriad of benefits for both physical and mental health, from reducing the risk of chronic diseases such as heart disease and diabetes to improving mood, cognition, and overall quality of life.

Yet, in our modern world, where sedentary lifestyles have become the norm, finding time for physical activity can be a challenge. We sit for hours on end, hunched over screens, our bodies growing stiff and sluggish with disuse. But the truth is, even small bursts of activity can make a world of difference.

Whether it's taking the stairs instead of the elevator, going for a walk during your lunch break, or practicing a few simple yoga poses before bed, every bit of movement counts.

The key is to find activities that you enjoy and that resonate with your body and spirit. Whether it's dancing, swimming, hiking, or practicing martial arts, there are countless ways to move your body and nourish your soul. Listen to your body's cues, and honor its need for rest and recovery as much as its need for movement and activity.

As you integrate physical activity into your daily routine, pay attention to how it makes you feel—not just physically, but emotionally and mentally as well. Notice the sense of lightness and vitality that comes from moving your body in ways that feel good and nourishing. Celebrate the small victories—the extra mile run, the deeper stretch, the feeling of strength and power coursing through your veins

In the pursuit of holistic wellness, physical activity serves as a cornerstone, anchoring us to the present moment and reminding us of the inherent vitality coursing through our veins. As we engage in movement, whether it's a brisk walk through nature's embrace or the rhythmic flow of a yoga practice, we become attuned to the symphony of sensations that animate our bodies.

Each movement is an act of self-love, a testament to our commitment to nurturing and honoring the vessel that carries us through life's journey. With each step, each stretch, each breath, we cultivate a deeper sense of connection to ourselves and the world around us.

But physical activity is not just about the physical; it is also a powerful tool for cultivating mental clarity and emotional resilience. In the midst of a challenging workout, we learn to quiet the chatter of the mind and focus our attention on the present moment. We discover strength we never knew we had, both physically and mentally, as we push through barriers and overcome obstacles.

And in the aftermath of exertion, we find solace in the stillness that follows, a sense of peace and tranquility that permeates every fiber of our being. As the body releases tension and stress, the mind becomes clear and calm, and we are left with a profound sense of well-being that extends far beyond the confines of the workout.

As you embark on your journey of holistic wellness, let physical activity be your faithful companion, guiding you along the path with grace and strength. Embrace movement as a sacred practice, a celebration of the incredible gift of life that resides within you. And with each step, each breath, each beat of your heart, may you find yourself moving closer to the radiant vitality and profound sense of well-being that awaits you on the journey ahead.

Physical activity is not just something we do; it is an integral part of who we are—a celebration of the incredible capabilities of the human body and a testament to the profound connection between body, mind, and spirit. So lace up your shoes, roll out your mat, and step into the flow of movement, where every step is a step towards holistic wellness.

Chapter 4

Restoring Balance: Sleep and Relaxation Techniques

Imagine yourself lying on a soft bed, enveloped in a cocoon of warmth and comfort, the cares of the day melting away as you drift into a state of deep relaxation. Sleep, that sacred refuge of rest and rejuvenation, holds within its embrace the power to restore balance to our weary bodies and minds. In this chapter, we delve into the profound importance of sleep and explore a variety of relaxation techniques to help you cultivate a more peaceful and restful state of being.

Sleep is not merely a passive state of unconsciousness; it is a dynamic process essential for the maintenance of physical, mental, and emotional well-being. During sleep, the body undergoes a remarkable array of physiological processes, including tissue repair, hormone regulation, and memory consolidation. It is during sleep that the brain sifts through the events of the day, integrating new information and experiences into our neural networks, and preparing us for the challenges that lie ahead.

Yet, in our fast-paced modern world, sleep is often treated as a luxury rather than a necessity. We push ourselves to the brink of exhaustion, sacrificing precious hours of rest in pursuit of productivity and achievement. But the truth is, sleep deprivation exacts a heavy toll on our health and well-being, impairing cognitive function, weakening the immune system, and increasing the risk of chronic disease.

So how can we reclaim the gift of restful sleep and restore balance to our lives? The journey begins with cultivating healthy sleep habits, known as sleep hygiene. This involves creating a conducive sleep environment, establishing a regular sleep schedule, and engaging in relaxing bedtime rituals to signal to the body that it is time to wind down.

One powerful relaxation technique that can promote restful sleep is deep breathing. By slowing down the breath and focusing on the rhythmic rise and fall of the chest, we can activate the body's relaxation response, signaling to the nervous system that it is safe to relax and unwind. Another effective technique is progressive muscle relaxation, which involves systematically tensing and releasing each muscle group in the body, allowing tension to melt away and paving the way for a more peaceful slumber.

In addition to these techniques, practices such as meditation, gentle yoga, and aromatherapy can also be valuable allies in the quest for better sleep. By quieting the mind, soothing the senses, and releasing physical tension, these practices can help us let go of the stresses of the day and sink into a state of deep relaxation.

One key aspect of restoring balance to your sleep is creating a sleep-friendly environment. This means minimizing exposure to stimulating activities and electronic devices before bedtime, dimming the lights, and creating a comfortable and tranquil atmosphere in your bedroom. Consider investing in a supportive mattress and pillows, as well as blackout curtains or a white noise machine to block out distractions and promote a deeper sleep.

Establishing a consistent sleep schedule can also play a significant role in improving sleep quality. Aim to go to bed and wake up at the same time each day, even on weekends, to regulate your body's internal clock and promote a more restful sleep-wake cycle. Avoiding caffeine, alcohol, and heavy meals close to bedtime can also help to facilitate better sleep by minimizing disruptions to your body's natural sleep rhythms.

In addition to creating a conducive sleep environment and maintaining a regular sleep schedule, it's important to engage in relaxing bedtime rituals to signal to your body that it is time to unwind. This could include activities such as taking a warm bath, practicing gentle yoga or stretching exercises, or reading a book before bed. Find activities that help you to relax and unwind, and incorporate them into your nightly routine to prepare your body and mind for sleep.

As you explore different relaxation techniques and bedtime rituals, pay attention to how they make you feel and how they impact your sleep quality. Keep a sleep journal to track your sleep patterns and any changes you notice in your sleep habits, and adjust your routine as needed to find what works best for you.

In addition to incorporating relaxation techniques into your bedtime routine, consider integrating moments of rest and rejuvenation into your daily life as well. This could involve taking short breaks throughout the day to pause, breathe deeply, and reconnect with yourself, allowing you to release tension and recharge your energy.

Moreover, be mindful of the role that stress and lifestyle factors may play in disrupting your sleep patterns. Chronic stress, busy schedules, and unhealthy habits can all contribute to sleep disturbances and undermine your efforts to restore balance. Take proactive steps to manage stress through practices such as mindfulness meditation, journaling, or spending time in nature. Prioritize self-care activities that nourish your body, mind, and spirit, such as exercise, healthy eating, and spending time with loved ones.

As you cultivate a deeper awareness of your sleep and relaxation needs, remember to approach this journey with compassion and kindness toward yourself. Be gentle with yourself during times of struggle, and celebrate your progress, no matter how small. Embrace the process of self-discovery and growth, knowing that each step you take brings you closer to a life filled with vitality, joy, and well-being.

Ultimately, the journey to restoring balance to your sleep and relaxation practices is a deeply personal one. It requires patience, self-awareness, and a willingness to prioritize your well-being. By nurturing a deeper connection to your body's natural rhythms and honoring its need for rest and rejuvenation, you can cultivate a greater sense of peace, vitality, and harmony in your life.

In conclusion, restoring balance to your sleep and relaxation practices is a journey of self-care and self-discovery that requires dedication, patience, and mindfulness. By prioritizing your sleep and embracing relaxation techniques, you can create a sanctuary of rest and rejuvenation in your life, allowing you to thrive and flourish in mind, body, and spirit.

Chapter 5

Emotions are the vibrant colors that paint the canvas of our lives, enriching our experiences, and shaping our perceptions of the world around us. Yet, like the ebb and flow of the tide, they can also carry us on tumultuous waves, leaving us feeling lost and adrift. In this chapter, we delve into the intricate landscape of emotional well-being, exploring the nuances of our feelings and learning how to cultivate a deeper sense of resilience, balance, and inner peace.

At the heart of emotional well-being lies the art of self-awareness—the ability to recognize, acknowledge, and honor our emotions without judgment or resistance. It is the willingness to sit with discomfort, to explore the depths of our feelings, and to embrace the full spectrum of our emotional landscape. Through mindfulness practices such as meditation and breathwork, we learn to cultivate a spacious awareness that allows us to observe our thoughts and emotions with curiosity and compassion.

Central to the practice of emotional well-being is the cultivation of emotional intelligence—the ability to navigate and regulate our emotions effectively. This involves developing skills such as self-awareness, self-regulation, empathy, and social skills, which enable us to navigate the complexities of interpersonal relationships with grace and understanding.

One of the cornerstones of emotional well-being is the practice of self-care—the act of nurturing ourselves on a physical, emotional, and spiritual level. This may involve engaging in activities that bring us joy and fulfillment, setting healthy boundaries, and prioritizing our own needs and well-being.

Another essential aspect of emotional well-being is the cultivation of healthy coping mechanisms for managing stress and adversity. This may involve practices such as journaling, creative expression, or spending time in nature, which provide outlets for processing and releasing pent-up emotions in a healthy and constructive manner.

Furthermore, fostering meaningful connections and relationships with others is crucial for emotional well-being. By cultivating authentic connections based on trust, empathy, and mutual support, we create a sense of belonging and interconnectedness that nourishes our emotional selves and strengthens our resilience in the face of life's challenges.

In our journey towards emotional well-being, it is important to remember that healing is not linear. There will be moments of struggle and setback, moments when we feel overwhelmed by the intensity of our emotions. In these moments, it is important to practice self-compassion—to extend kindness and understanding to ourselves, knowing that our emotions are a natural and integral part of the human experience.

As we deepen our understanding of ourselves and our emotions, we may uncover layers of complexity and nuance that were previously hidden from view. This unfolding journey invites us to approach our emotional landscape with curiosity, openness, and a willingness to learn and grow.

Within the path of emotional well-being, there exists a rich variety of practices and techniques that can support us on our journey. Mindfulness-based approaches, such as mindfulness meditation and mindful movement, offer powerful tools for cultivating present-moment awareness and cultivating a sense of inner peace amidst life's challenges.

Additionally, techniques such as cognitive-behavioral therapy (CBT) and dialectical behavior therapy (DBT) provide practical strategies for identifying and challenging unhelpful thought patterns and behaviors, fostering greater emotional resilience and well-being.

Exploring our creativity can also be a potent pathway to emotional healing and self-expression. Engaging in creative pursuits such as art, music, writing, or dance can provide a safe and sacred space for exploring and processing our emotions, allowing us to tap into our inner wisdom and express ourselves authentically.

Moreover, the practice of self-compassion is essential for nurturing emotional well-being. By treating ourselves with kindness, acceptance, and understanding, even in the midst of difficult emotions, we cultivate a sense of inner warmth and resilience that can carry us through life's challenges with grace and compassion.

As we navigate the terrain of emotional well-being, it's important to remember that we are not alone on this journey. Seeking support from trusted friends, family members, or mental health professionals can provide invaluable guidance, validation, and encouragement along the way.

Ultimately, the journey towards emotional well-being is a deeply personal and transformative process—one that invites us to embrace the fullness of our humanity and to cultivate a deep sense of compassion, resilience, and inner peace. By tending to our emotional selves with care and compassion, we can create a life that is rich in meaning, connection, and fulfillment, grounded in the deep knowing that we are worthy of love and belonging just as we are.

Chapter 6

Harnessing the Power of Mindfulness and Meditation

In the busy chaos of modern life, our minds often resemble a turbulent sea, tossed about by the waves of thoughts, emotions, and distractions. Yet, amidst this storm, there exists an oasis of calm—a sanctuary within each of us where we can find refuge from the tumult of the outside world. This sanctuary is mindfulness and meditation, ancient practices that have stood the test of time as powerful tools for cultivating inner peace, clarity, and presence.

Mindfulness, simply put, is the practice of being fully present in the moment, with awareness and acceptance of our thoughts, feelings, sensations, and surroundings. It is about bringing our attention to the here and now, without judgment or attachment, allowing us to experience life with greater clarity, insight, and equanimity.

Meditation, on the other hand, is the intentional cultivation of mindfulness through various techniques and practices, such as focused attention, breath awareness, loving-kindness, and body scan meditation. These practices offer us a way to quiet the incessant chatter of the mind, to drop beneath the surface of our thoughts and emotions, and to tap into the deep wellspring of peace and wisdom that lies within.

As we embark on the journey of mindfulness and meditation, it's important to approach these practices with an open mind and a spirit of curiosity and exploration. There is no one-size-fits-all approach to mindfulness and meditation, and what works for one person may not resonate with another. It's about finding the techniques and practices that resonate most deeply with us and incorporating them into our daily lives in a way that feels authentic and sustainable.

One of the simplest and most accessible forms of meditation is breath awareness meditation. To practice, find a quiet and comfortable space where you can sit or lie down without distractions. Close your eyes and bring your attention to your breath, noticing the sensation of the breath as it enters and leaves your body. You may choose to focus on the rise and fall of your chest or the sensation of air passing through your nostrils. Whenever your mind begins to wander—which it inevitably will—simply gently guide your attention back to your breath, without judgment or frustration.

Another powerful meditation practice is loving-kindness meditation, also known as metta meditation. This practice involves cultivating feelings of love, compassion, and goodwill towards ourselves and others. To practice, begin by bringing to mind someone for whom you have deep love and affection—this could be a friend, family member, or even a beloved pet. Silently repeat phrases of loving-kindness towards this person, such as "May you be happy, may you be healthy, may you be safe, may you be at ease." As you continue, gradually expand the circle of loving-kindness to include yourself, then to acquaintances, and finally to all beings everywhere.

Mindfulness and meditation are not quick fixes or magic bullets; they are lifelong practices that require patience, dedication, and commitment. Like tending to a garden, they require regular care and attention in order to flourish and bear fruit. But with time and practice, the fruits of mindfulness and meditation—peace, clarity, and presence—will ripen within us, enriching every aspect of our lives and illuminating the path to holistic wellness.

Incorporating mindfulness and meditation into our daily lives can have profound effects on our physical, mental, and emotional well-being. Research has shown that regular mindfulness and meditation practice can reduce stress, anxiety, and depression, while enhancing resilience, focus, and emotional regulation.

Beyond the individual benefits, mindfulness and meditation also have ripple effects that extend outward, influencing our relationships, our communities, and the world at large. When we cultivate inner peace and compassion within ourselves, we become more capable of extending that peace and compassion to others, fostering greater empathy, understanding, and connection in our interactions with those around us.

Moreover, mindfulness and meditation can serve as powerful tools for social and environmental change, helping us to cultivate the awareness, compassion, and resilience needed to navigate the challenges of our times with grace and wisdom. As we become more attuned to the interconnectedness of all beings and the interdependence of life on Earth, we are inspired to act with greater kindness, compassion, and stewardship towards ourselves, each other, and the planet.

But perhaps the greatest gift of mindfulness and meditation is the profound sense of presence and aliveness that they bring to our lives. In a world that often feels fragmented and disconnected, mindfulness and meditation offer us a way to come home to ourselves, to reconnect with the deep wellspring of peace, wisdom, and joy that lies within each of us.

As we continue on the journey of mindfulness and meditation, may we remember that the path is not always smooth or linear. There will be days when our minds feel scattered and restless, when our hearts feel heavy and burdened. But even in the midst of the storm, we can take refuge in the sanctuary of mindfulness and meditation, returning again and again to the present moment with gentle kindness and compassion.

In the end, it is not the destination that matters, but the journey itself—the moments of stillness and silence, the breaths taken with mindful awareness, the heart opening to the vastness of existence. In these moments, we glimpse the infinite possibilities that lie within us, and we remember that true happiness and fulfillment are not found in the external world, but in the depths of our own being.

So let us continue on this journey with open hearts and open minds, embracing each moment with curiosity and wonder, knowing that every step we take brings us closer to the radiant vitality and profound sense of well-being that awaits us at the journey's end.

Chapter 7

Exploring Alternative Healing Modalities

As we delve deeper into the realm of holistic wellness, we encounter a rich tapestry of alternative healing modalities, each offering its own unique approach to supporting health and well-being. In this chapter, we will explore several of these modalities in depth, shedding light on their principles, practices, and potential benefits.

Acupuncture:

Originating in ancient China thousands of years ago, acupuncture is a key component of traditional Chinese medicine (TCM). At its core is the belief that the body is traversed by a network of channels, or meridians, through which vital energy, known as Qi, flows. When these channels become blocked or imbalanced, it can lead to illness and discomfort. Acupuncture aims to restore balance and promote healing by inserting thin needles into specific points along the meridians, stimulating the body's natural healing mechanisms and restoring the flow of Qi.

Acupuncture is a cornerstone of traditional Chinese medicine (TCM), rooted in the belief that the body is traversed by a network of meridians through which vital energy, or Qi, flows. When this flow is disrupted or blocked, it can lead to illness and discomfort. Acupuncture involves the insertion of thin needles into specific points along these meridians to stimulate the body's natural healing mechanisms and restore balance. The needles may be manipulated manually or stimulated with heat or electricity to enhance their effects. Acupuncture is used to treat a wide range of conditions, including chronic pain,stress, anxiety, digestive disorders, and reproductive issues.

Herbal Medicine:

Herbal medicine is one of the oldest forms of healing, with roots dating back to ancient civilizations around the world. It harnesses the therapeutic properties of plants to prevent and treat a wide range of ailments. Herbs are used in various forms, including teas, tinctures, extracts, and topical preparations. Each herb contains a complex array of chemical compounds that interact with the body in unique ways, offering benefits such as anti-inflammatory, antimicrobial, and antioxidant effects. Herbal medicine is often used in conjunction with other holistic modalities to support overall health and well-being.

Herbal medicine, also known as botanical medicine or phytotherapy, utilizes the therapeutic properties of plants to prevent and treat illness. Herbs contain a complex array of chemical compounds, including alkaloids, flavonoids, and terpenes, which interact with the body in unique ways. Herbal remedies can be prepared in various forms, such as teas, tinctures, capsules, and topical preparations. Each herb has specific actions and indications, and herbalists carefully select and combine herbs to address individual needs and health concerns. Herbal medicine is used to support a wide range of health issues, from acute infections and chronic diseases to emotional imbalances and general wellness maintenance

Energy Healing:

Energy healing encompasses a diverse range of practices that work with the body's subtle energy systems to promote healing and balance. One such modality is Reiki, a Japanese technique that channels universal life force energy to support healing on physical, emotional, and spiritual levels. During a Reiki session, the practitioner places their hands on or near the client's body, allowing the energy to flow through them and into the recipient. This gentle yet powerful energy helps to dissolve energetic blockages, promote relaxation, and enhance the body's natural healing abilities.

Energy healing encompasses a diverse range of practices that work with the body's subtle energy systems to promote healing and balance. These modalities are based on the understanding that everything in the universe, including our bodies, is composed of energy vibrating at different frequencies. By working with these subtle energies, energy healers can help to remove energetic blockages, restore balance, and facilitate healing on physical, emotional, and spiritual levels. Techniques such as Reiki, Healing Touch, and Pranic Healing involve channeling or manipulating energy to promote relaxation,reduce pain, boost the immune system, and enhance overall well-being.

Homeopathy:

Homeopathy is a holistic system of medicine founded in the late 18th century by German physician Samuel Hahnemann. It is based on the principle of "like cures like," which states that a substance that produces symptoms in a healthy person can be used to treat similar symptoms in a sick person when diluted to minute doses. Homeopathic remedies are prepared through a process of serial dilution and succussion, which is believed to enhance their healing properties while minimizing side effects. Homeopathy is used to address a wide range of physical, emotional, and mental health issues and is tailored to each individual's unique constitution.

Sound Healing:

Sound healing is an ancient practice that utilizes the power of sound vibrations to promote healing and relaxation. It draws on the understanding that everything in the universe, including our bodies, is in a state of vibration. By exposing the body to specific frequencies and rhythms, sound healing can help to entrain the body's own vibrations to a state of harmony and balance. Modalities such as Tibetan singing bowls, crystal bowls, tuning forks, and vocal toning are used to generate healing frequencies that resonate with different aspects of the body and psyche.

By exposing the body to specific frequencies and rhythms, sound healing can help to entrain the body's own vibrations to a state of harmony and balance. Modalities such as Tibetan singing bowls, crystal bowls, tuning forks, and vocal toning are used to generate healing frequencies that resonate with different aspects of the body and psyche. Sound healing is used to reduce stress, alleviate pain, improve sleep, enhance concentration, and facilitate spiritual growth and transformation.

As we explore these alternative healing modalities, it is important to approach them with an open mind and a spirit of curiosity. While they may seem unconventional to some, they have stood the test of time and continue to offer profound benefits to those who seek them out. Whether used alone or in conjunction with conventional medicine, these modalities have the potential to support holistic wellness and enhance our quality of life in profound and meaningful ways.

Crystal Healing:

Crystal healing is based on the belief that crystals and gemstones possess unique vibrational properties that can help to balance and align the body's energy systems. Each crystal is thought to resonate with specific energy centers, or chakras, within the body, and can be used to address imbalances and promote healing. Crystals can be placed on or around the body during a session, or worn as jewelry or carried in a pocket for ongoing support. They are believed to absorb, store, and transmit energy, helping to restore harmony and vitality to the mind, body, and spirit.

Aromatherapy:

Aromatherapy is the practice of using essential oils extracted from plants to promote physical, emotional, and spiritual well-being. These potent oils contain the concentrated essence of the plant, including its aromatic compounds and therapeutic properties. Inhalation, topical application, and diffusion are common methods of using essential oils, each offering unique benefits. For example, inhaling the scent of lavender oil can promote relaxation and reduce stress, while applying peppermint oil to the skin can alleviate headaches and improve mental clarity. Aromatherapy is often used in conjunction with massage, meditation, and other holistic practices to enhance their effects.

Massage Therapy:

Massage therapy is a hands-on healing modality that has been practiced for thousands of years in cultures around the world. It involves manipulating the soft tissues of the body, such as muscles, tendons, and ligaments, to promote relaxation, reduce tension, and relieve pain. Various massage techniques, including Swedish massage, deep tissue massage, and shiatsu, target different areas of the body and address specific concerns. In addition to its physical benefits, massage therapy also has profound effects on mental and emotional well-being, helping to reduce anxiety, depression, and stress.

Holistic Nutrition:

Holistic nutrition is a comprehensive approach to eating that takes into account the interconnectedness of food, health, and well-being. It emphasizes the importance of eating whole, nutrient-dense foods that nourish the body and support optimal function. Holistic nutritionists consider not only the nutritional content of foods, but also their energetic properties, environmental impact, and cultural significance. They work with clients to develop personalized nutrition plans that address their unique needs and goals, taking into account factors such as food sensitivities, digestive health, and emotional eating patterns.

As we explore these alternative healing modalities, we gain a deeper appreciation for the diverse ways in which we can support our health and well-being. Each modality offers its own unique approach to healing, yet they all share a common goal: to help us reconnect with our innate capacity for health, vitality, and wholeness. By embracing the wisdom of these ancient practices and integrating them into our lives, we can unlock the full potential of holistic wellness and embark on a journey of self-discovery, healing, and transformation.

Chapter 8

Creating Harmonious Environments

As we delve into the realm of holistic wellness, we come to understand that our external environment plays a profound role in shaping our inner landscape. Just as the quality of the soil determines the health of a plant, the spaces we inhabit can either nourish or deplete our vitality, influencing our physical, mental, and emotional well-being in profound ways.

Our homes, workplaces, and the natural world that surrounds us are not merely physical spaces but living, breathing ecosystems that interact with our own energetic fields. When these environments are in harmony with our own energy, they can support and enhance our well-being. Conversely, when they are out of alignment, they can create discord and imbalance, sapping our energy and vitality.

Creating harmonious environments begins with cultivating awareness of the subtle energies that permeate our surroundings. Just as we tune into the rhythms of our own bodies, we must learn to attune ourselves to the energy of the spaces we inhabit, listening to the whispers of the wind, feeling the warmth of the sun on our skin, and sensing the pulse of life that animates all things.

One of the fundamental principles of creating harmonious environments is the concept of Feng Shui, an ancient Chinese practice that seeks to harmonize the flow of energy, or chi, in our living and working spaces. According to Feng Shui principles, the layout, design, and arrangement of our environments can either facilitate the smooth flow of chi or create blockages and stagnation.

By applying Feng Shui principles to our homes and workplaces, we can optimize the flow of energy, creating spaces that feel balanced, harmonious, and supportive of our well-being. This may involve arranging furniture to promote the free flow of energy, incorporating natural elements such as plants and water features, and decluttering our spaces to remove obstacles that impede the flow of chi.

In addition to Feng Shui, there are numerous other practices and techniques we can use to create harmonious environments. Mindfulness, for example, teaches us to be fully present in the moment, allowing us to appreciate the beauty and sacredness of our surroundings. By bringing mindfulness to our environments, we can infuse even the most mundane spaces with a sense of wonder and reverence.

Another powerful practice for creating harmonious environments is the use of sacred rituals and ceremonies. Whether it's lighting a candle, smudging with sage, or setting intentions for the space, these rituals can help us to imbue our environments with positive energy and intention, creating a sense of sacredness and reverence.

Another aspect of creating harmonious environments involves the conscious selection of materials and objects that resonate with our energy and values. Just as certain foods nourish our bodies more effectively than others, certain materials and objects carry energetic vibrations that can either uplift or drain our energy.

Choosing natural, sustainable materials such as wood, stone, and organic fabrics can help to create environments that feel grounded, nourishing, and in harmony with the natural world. Similarly, surrounding ourselves with objects that hold personal significance or evoke positive emotions can infuse our spaces with a sense of warmth, comfort, and joy.

However, creating harmonious environments is not solely about the physical aspects of our surroundings; it also involves cultivating healthy boundaries and relationships within our social and interpersonal environments. Just as toxic chemicals can pollute the air we breathe, toxic relationships can poison our emotional and energetic well-being.

Learning to set boundaries, communicate assertively, and surround ourselves with people who uplift and support us are essential components of creating harmonious social environments. By surrounding ourselves with individuals who respect and honor our boundaries, we can create relationships that nourish and sustain us, fostering a sense of connection, belonging, and community.

Finally, creating harmonious environments is an ongoing practice—a journey rather than a destination. Just as the seasons change and evolve, so too do our environments, and it is up to us to adapt and evolve along with them. By remaining mindful and attentive to the ever-changing rhythms of life, we can continue to cultivate environments that support and enhance our well-being, nurturing the seeds of harmony, balance, and vitality within ourselves and the world around us..

Chapter 9

Connecting with Nature

Imagine yourself standing on the edge of a rugged cliff, the salty breeze caressing your skin and the roar of the ocean filling your ears. Before you stretches a vast expanse of untouched wilderness, teeming with life and brimming with beauty. This is nature in all its untamed glory—a sanctuary for the soul, a refuge from the chaos of modern life.

Nature has a way of calling to us, beckoning us to step outside the confines of our daily routines and reconnect with the natural world. It is in nature that we find solace, inspiration, and a profound sense of belonging. But in our fast-paced, technology-driven world, it is all too easy to lose touch with the healing power of nature and the deep connection it offers us.

To truly connect with nature is to immerse ourselves in its rhythms and cycles, to tune into its subtle sounds and profound wisdom. It is to recognize that we are not separate from nature, but intrinsically intertwined with it—a part of the intricate web of life that spans the globe.

As you step into the embrace of nature, allow yourself to surrender to its beauty and majesty. Feel the soft earth beneath your feet, grounding you and anchoring you to the present moment. Listen to the symphony of sounds that fills the air—the chirping of birds, the rustling of leaves, the gentle lapping of waves against the shore. Let these sounds wash over you, soothing your soul and quieting your mind.

Take a deep breath and inhale the fragrant scent of the forest, the salty tang of the sea, the crisp freshness of the mountain air. Let the aromas of nature awaken your senses and invigorate your spirit, filling you with a sense of vitality and aliveness.

As you move through nature, allow yourself to be fully present in each moment, allowing the sights, sounds, and sensations to wash over you like a cleansing wave. Notice the intricate beauty of a flower in bloom, the graceful dance of a butterfly on the breeze, the silent majesty of a towering redwood tree. Let these moments of awe and wonder fill you with gratitude and reverence for the natural world.

But connecting with nature is not just about being in its presence; it is about forging a deep and meaningful relationship with the earth and all its inhabitants. It is about honoring the earth as a sacred and sentient being, deserving of our love, respect, and protection.

As you deepen your connection with nature, consider ways in which you can give back to the earth and contribute to its healing and restoration. Whether it's planting a tree, cleaning up a beach, or supporting conservation efforts in your community, every act of kindness and stewardship helps to nurture and preserve the precious gift of nature for generations to come.

In this journey of connecting with nature, let us explore the diverse landscapes that adorn our planet, each offering its own unique gifts and teachings. Venture into the heart of lush forests, where ancient trees stand sentinel, their roots intertwined with the wisdom of the ages. Wander along winding trails that lead to hidden waterfalls, their cascading waters a symphony of serenity and renewal.

As you explore nature's wonders, take the time to cultivate a sense of awe and wonder for the intricate ecosystems that sustain life on Earth. Marvel at the delicate balance of flora and fauna, each species playing its part in the grand symphony of creation. Witness the interconnectedness of all living things, as plants breathe life into the air we breathe, and animals shape the landscapes they inhabit.

But connecting with nature is not just about awe-inspiring landscapes and majestic vistas—it is also about finding beauty and wonder in the smallest of details. Pause to admire the intricate patterns of a leaf, the delicate petals of a flower, the graceful flight of a butterfly. Let these moments of quiet observation awaken your sense of wonder and deepen your appreciation for the beauty and complexity of the natural world.

As you immerse yourself in the healing embrace of nature, allow yourself to be transformed by its profound wisdom and nurturing presence. Let go of the stresses and worries of daily life, and surrender to the tranquility and peace that nature offers. Allow its rhythms to synchronize with your own, restoring harmony and balance to mind, body, and spirit.

In the end, connecting with nature is about more than just finding moments of solace and serenity—it is about forging a deep and intimate relationship with the earth and all its inhabitants. It is about recognizing that we are not separate from nature, but deeply interconnected with it, and that our well-being is intricately linked to the health and vitality of the planet.

So let us embrace the call of nature, and embark on a journey of discovery, connection, and reverence for the natural world that sustains us all. For in nature, we find not only beauty and inspiration, but also the wisdom and healing power to nourish our souls and transform our lives.

Chapter 10

Developing Spiritual Practices

In the labyrinth of holistic wellness, one of the most profound and transformative paths lies in the exploration of spiritual practices. As we delve into this realm, we encounter the essence of our being—the spark of divinity that resides within each of us, waiting to be awakened and nurtured.

Spirituality is a deeply personal journey, unique to each individual, yet it is also a universal language that transcends cultural boundaries and religious beliefs. At its core, spirituality is about cultivating a sense of connection—to ourselves, to others, to the natural world, and to something

greater than ourselves. It is about finding meaning and purpose in our lives, and tapping into a source of wisdom and guidance that transcends the limitations of our finite minds.
Central to the practice of spirituality is the cultivation of presence—the art of being fully present in each moment, without judgment or attachment. This requires us to quiet the chatter of our minds and attune ourselves to the subtle whispers of our souls. Through practices such as meditation, prayer, and mindfulness, we learn to quiet the noise of the external world and listen to the wisdom that resides within.

Meditation, perhaps the most well-known spiritual practice, offers a gateway into the depths of our inner being. Through the simple act of sitting in stillness and silence, we cultivate a deep sense of peace and tranquility, allowing us to connect with the essence of our being. In the silence of meditation, we may encounter insights, revelations, and profound states of bliss that transcend the limitations of our ordinary consciousness.

Prayer, another cornerstone of spiritual practice, is a means of connecting with the divine—the source of all creation. Whether we address our prayers to a specific deity, the universe, or our own inner wisdom, prayer is a powerful tool for expressing gratitude, seeking guidance, and offering up our hopes, fears, and aspirations.

Mindfulness, perhaps the most accessible of spiritual practices, invites us to bring a sense of presence and awareness to every moment of our lives. By cultivating mindfulness in our daily activities—whether eating, walking,

or simply breathing—we can experience a profound sense of aliveness and connectedness to the world around us.
Beyond the realms of meditation, prayer, and mindfulness lies a vast landscape of spiritual practices waiting to be explored. Among them, the practice of yoga stands as a sign of union, inviting us to unite body, mind, and spirit in a dance of breath and movement.

Yoga, derived from the Sanskrit word "yuj," meaning to yoke or unite, offers a holistic approach to wellness that encompasses physical postures (asanas), breathwork (pranayama), meditation, and philosophical teachings. Through the practice of yoga, we cultivate strength, flexibility, and balance in both body and mind, while deepening our connection to the divine within and without.

In the embrace of nature, we find yet another avenue for spiritual exploration and connection. Whether it be a solitary walk in the woods, a sunrise meditation by the ocean, or simply sitting beneath the canopy of a tree, nature offers us a sanctuary—a sacred space in which to commune with the natural world and the universal forces that animate it.

Sacred rituals and ceremonies, passed down through generations, offer us a means of honoring the cycles of nature, the rhythms of life, and the milestones of our own journeys. Whether it be a simple daily ritual of lighting a candle and offering a prayer of gratitude, or a more elaborate ceremony marking a significant life event, rituals serve as potent reminders of the sacredness of life and our interconnectedness with all of creation.

In the realm of creative expression, we discover yet another pathway to the divine. Whether through art, music, dance, or poetry, creative expression allows us to tap into the boundless wellspring of inspiration that lies within, channeling the energy of the cosmos into tangible form.

As we journey deeper into the realm of spiritual practice, we may encounter challenges and obstacles along the way. Doubt, fear, and resistance may arise, tempting us to turn back or seek refuge in familiar comforts. Yet it is precisely in these moments of challenge that our spiritual practice becomes most potent, serving as a beacon of light to guide us through the darkness and into the luminous depths of our own being.

In the practice of spirituality, there are no shortcuts or quick fixes—only the invitation to journey deeper into the mystery of existence, to embrace the fullness of our humanity, and to awaken to the divine light that shines within us all. And as we walk this path of self-discovery and self-transformation, may we find solace, strength, and inspiration in the knowledge that we are never alone—that we are part of a vast and interconnected web of beings, all walking this journey together toward the radiant dawn of awakening.

In addition to these core practices, there are countless other spiritual practices that we may explore on our journey of self-discovery and self-transformation. From yoga and tai chi to chanting and sacred rituals, the possibilities are as vast and varied as the human spirit itself.

As we embark on the path of spiritual practice, it is important to approach with openness, curiosity, and a willingness to explore the depths of our own being. There is no one-size-fits-all approach to spirituality, and what works for one person may not resonate with another. The key is to listen to the whispers of our hearts, follow our intuition, and trust in the wisdom of our own inner guidance.

In the practice of spirituality, there are no rigid rules or dogmas to follow—only the invitation to explore, to experiment, and to discover the sacred within ourselves and the world around us. And as we journey deeper into the realm of the spirit, may we find solace, strength, and inspiration to guide us on our path to holistic wellness.

Chapter 11

Integrating Holistic Wellness into Daily Life

As we delve into the heart of holistic wellness, we encounter the profound challenge of integrating its principles into our daily lives. It's not enough to simply understand the concepts; we must embody them in our thoughts, actions, and interactions with the world around us. In this chapter, we explore practical strategies for weaving the threads of holistic wellness into the fabric of our daily existence.

Morning Rituals:

The morning sets the tone for the rest of the day, making it an ideal time to cultivate holistic wellness practices. Begin by greeting the day with gratitude, acknowledging the gift of another opportunity for growth and transformation. Engage in gentle movement or stretching to awaken the body and invigorate the mind. Set intentions for the day ahead, aligning them with your values and aspirations. And nourish yourself with a wholesome breakfast, fueling your body for the challenges and joys that lie ahead.

Mindful Living:

At its core, holistic wellness is about living with intention and awareness, bringing mindfulness to every moment of our lives. Practice mindfulness in everyday activities, such as eating, walking, and interacting with others. Cultivate present-moment awareness, savoring the richness of each experience without judgment or attachment. And carve out moments of stillness and silence amidst the busyness of daily life, allowing yourself to reconnect with your innermost self and the wisdom that resides within.

Nutrition and Diet:

The foods we consume have a profound impact on our physical, mental, and emotional well-being. Embrace a whole foods-based diet rich in fruits, vegetables, whole grains, and lean proteins, nourishing your body with the nutrients it needs to thrive. Practice mindful eating, savoring each bite and paying attention to your body's hunger and fullness cues. And cultivate a healthy relationship with food, free from guilt, shame, or restriction, honoring your body's unique needs and preferences.

Movement and Exercise:

Physical activity is essential for supporting optimal health and vitality, but it need not be a chore. Find joy in movement by exploring activities that bring you pleasure and fulfillment, whether it's dancing, hiking, yoga, or simply taking a leisurely stroll in nature. Listen to your body's cues and honor its limitations, choosing activities that feel nourishing and supportive rather than punitive or draining. And remember that movement is not just about burning calories; it's about celebrating the incredible capabilities of your body and reveling in the joy of being alive.

Connection and Community:

Human connection is a fundamental aspect of holistic wellness, nourishing our souls and fostering a sense of belonging and purpose. Cultivate meaningful relationships with friends, family, and community members, nurturing connections that uplift and inspire you. Practice empathy, compassion, and active listening in your interactions with others, fostering deep bonds of understanding and support. And remember that true connection begins with yourself; honor your own needs and boundaries, and approach relationships with authenticity and vulnerability.

Self-Care and Stress Management:

In the fast-paced world we inhabit, self-care is often overlooked or neglected, yet it is essential for maintaining balance and well-being. Prioritize self-care by carving out time for activities that replenish and rejuvenate you, whether it's reading a book, taking a bath, or practicing meditation. Set boundaries around your time and energy, saying no to commitments that drain you and yes to those that nourish you. And develop effective stress management strategies, such as deep breathing, progressive muscle relaxation, or spending time in nature, to help you navigate life's inevitable challenges with grace and resilience.

Evening Reflections:

As the day draws to a close, take time to reflect on the events and experiences that unfolded. Practice gratitude for the blessings you received and the lessons you learned, acknowledging the beauty and complexity of life's journey. Release any lingering tensions or worries through gentle movement, breathwork, or journaling, allowing yourself to enter into a state of deep relaxation and ease. And set intentions for the night ahead, cultivating a sense of peace and serenity that will carry you into restful sleep and prepare you for the new day to come.

Integrating holistic wellness into daily life is not a one-time endeavor; it is an ongoing practice that requires commitment, dedication, and self-awareness. By weaving the threads of holistic wellness into the fabric of our daily existence, we can create a life of greater balance, vitality, and meaning. And as we embrace this journey with open hearts and open minds, may we discover the profound beauty and joy that awaits us in every moment.

Sustainability and Flexibility:

One of the keys to successfully integrating holistic wellness into daily life is to approach it with a mindset of sustainability and flexibility. Recognize that wellness is not a rigid set of rules to be followed dogmatically, but rather a dynamic and evolving journey that adapts to the changing rhythms of life. Be gentle with yourself when setbacks occur, and embrace imperfection as a natural part of the process. Cultivate a sense of curiosity and openness, allowing yourself to explore new practices and adapt existing ones to better suit your needs and circumstances.

Creating Rituals and Routines:

Rituals and routines can provide structure and stability in our lives, anchoring us in the present moment and grounding us amidst the chaos of daily life. Identify activities that bring you joy, peace, and fulfillment, and incorporate them into your daily or weekly routines as sacred rituals. Whether it's a morning meditation practice, an evening gratitude journaling session, or a weekly nature walk, these rituals can serve as anchors that remind us of our commitment to holistic wellness and reconnect us with our deepest selves.

Mindful Technology Use:

In today's digital age, technology has become an integral part of our lives, offering unprecedented access to information, connection, and entertainment. However, excessive use of technology can also disrupt our well-being, leading to stress, distraction, and disconnection from ourselves and others. Practice mindful technology use by setting boundaries around your screen time, taking regular breaks to disconnect and recharge, and cultivating awareness of how technology affects your mental and emotional state. Use technology as a tool for enhancing your well-being, rather than allowing it to control or overwhelm you.

Cultivating Gratitude and Joy:

Gratitude and joy are powerful antidotes to stress, anxiety, and negativity, helping us cultivate a mindset of abundance and appreciation for the blessings in our lives. Cultivate gratitude by keeping a gratitude journal, regularly reflecting on the things you are thankful for, and expressing appreciation to those around you. Seek out moments of joy and beauty in everyday life, whether it's watching a sunrise, sharing a laugh with a loved one, or savoring a delicious meal. By nurturing gratitude and joy in our hearts, we can cultivate a deeper sense of well-being and resilience in the face of life's challenges.

Embracing Impermanence:

In our quest for holistic wellness, it's important to remember that life is inherently impermanent and ever-changing. Embrace the ebb and flow of life's rhythms, allowing yourself to surrender to the natural cycles of growth, decay, and renewal. Recognize that challenges and setbacks are inevitable, but they also offer opportunities for growth, learning, and transformation. Cultivate a sense of resilience and adaptability, trusting in your ability to navigate life's twists and turns with grace and equanimity. And remember that even in the midst of life's challenges, there is beauty to be found, if only we have eyes to see it.

Integrating holistic wellness into daily life is a deeply personal and individual journey, guided by our unique needs, values, and aspirations. As you embark on this journey, remember to be gentle with yourself, patient with your progress, and open to the infinite possibilities that await you. By weaving the threads of holistic wellness into the fabric of your daily existence, you can create a life of greater balance, vitality, and meaning—a life that honors the interconnectedness of all things and celebrates the profound beauty of the human experience.

Chapter 12

Overcoming Challenges and Obstacles

In the labyrinth of life, obstacles often emerge as formidable adversaries, casting shadows on our path to holistic wellness. Yet, it is within the crucible of challenge that our resilience is forged, and our capacity for growth is tested. In this chapter, we confront the myriad challenges and obstacles that may impede our journey towards well-being, exploring strategies to overcome them with grace and fortitude.

1. Identifying Inner Resistance: At times, our greatest obstacle lies within ourselves—in the form of self-doubt, fear, or limiting beliefs. By cultivating self-awareness and mindfulness, we can shine a light on these inner demons, acknowledging them without judgment and gradually loosening their grip on our psyche.

2. Navigating External Pressures: External pressures, whether from work, relationships, or societal expectations, can exert a powerful influence on our well-being. Learning to set boundaries, prioritize self-care, and communicate our needs effectively are essential skills for navigating these external pressures while staying true to our path.

3. Managing Stress and Burnout: In our fast-paced world, stress and burnout have become ubiquitous threats to our health and well-being. By adopting stress-management techniques such as deep breathing, meditation, and time management, we can cultivate resilience in the face of adversity and prevent burnout before it takes hold.

4. Overcoming Setbacks and Failures: Setbacks and failures are an inevitable part of the human experience, yet they can feel like insurmountable obstacles on our journey to wellness. By reframing setbacks as opportunities for growth and learning, we can extract valuable lessons from adversity and emerge stronger and more resilient than before.

5. Cultivating Patience and Perseverance: Rome wasn't built in a day, and neither is holistic wellness achieved overnight. Cultivating patience and perseverance is essential for navigating the inevitable ups and downs of the journey, staying committed to our goals, and trusting in the process of transformation.

6. Seeking Support and Community: No journey is meant to be traveled alone. Seeking support from friends, family, or a like-minded community can provide us with the encouragement, accountability, and solidarity we need to overcome challenges and stay the course.

7. Embracing Self-Compassion: In moments of struggle and adversity, self-compassion becomes our most potent ally. By treating ourselves with kindness, understanding, and forgiveness, we can soften the harsh edges of self-criticism and cultivate a deep sense of inner resilience and self-worth.

8. Embracing the Journey: Ultimately, holistic wellness is not a destination but a journey—a journey of self-discovery, growth, and transformation. Embracing the journey means embracing the full spectrum of human experience—the joys and the sorrows, the triumphs and the challenges—and finding beauty and meaning in every step along the way.

9. Cultivating Adaptive Coping Strategies: When faced with unexpected challenges or setbacks, having a repertoire of adaptive coping strategies can be invaluable. These may include problem-solving skills, reframing negative thoughts, seeking social support, or engaging in creative outlets such as journaling or art therapy. By developing flexibility in our approach to adversity, we can adapt more readily to changing circumstances and navigate challenges with greater ease.

10. Honoring Personal Boundaries: Establishing and maintaining healthy boundaries is essential for preserving our physical, emotional, and mental well-being. Whether it's saying no to additional commitments, setting limits on social media usage, or advocating for our needs in relationships, honoring our boundaries empowers us to prioritize self-care and protect our holistic wellness.

11. Finding Meaning in Adversity: While adversity may bring pain and discomfort, it also offers an opportunity for growth and transformation. By reframing challenges as opportunities for meaning-making and personal development, we can extract valuable lessons from even the most difficult experiences and emerge with a deeper sense of purpose and resilience.

12. Cultivating Resilience Through Mindfulness and Self-Compassion: Mindfulness and self-compassion are powerful tools for building resilience in the face of adversity. By cultivating present-moment awareness and treating ourselves with kindness and understanding, we can navigate life's challenges with greater equanimity and grace, bouncing back from setbacks with renewed strength and resilience.

13. Seeking Professional Support When Needed: In times of significant challenge or adversity, seeking professional support from a therapist, counselor, or healthcare provider can provide invaluable guidance, insight, and validation. Whether facing mental health struggles, navigating relationship difficulties, or coping with trauma, reaching out for professional support is a courageous act of self-care that can facilitate healing and growth.

14. Cultivating Gratitude and Optimism: Cultivating an attitude of gratitude and optimism can help shift our perspective on challenges, allowing us to see them as opportunities for growth and learning rather than insurmountable obstacles. By focusing on the blessings in our lives and maintaining a hopeful outlook for the future, we can cultivate resilience and navigate adversity with greater resilience and grace.

15. Embracing the Journey with Acceptance and Surrender: Ultimately, overcoming challenges and obstacles on the path to holistic wellness requires a willingness to embrace the journey with acceptance and surrender. Accepting life's inevitable ups and downs, surrendering to the flow of change, and trusting in the inherent wisdom of the universe can help us find peace and resilience in the face of adversity, guiding us ever closer to the radiant vitality and profound well-being that await us on the other side.

..

Chapter 13

Sustaining Long-Term Wellness

As we journey through life, navigating its twists and turns, we inevitably encounter moments of triumph and challenge, joy and sorrow. Along the path of holistic wellness, these moments serve as signposts, guiding us toward greater understanding and deeper connection with ourselves and the world around us. we delve into the essential principles of sustaining long-term wellness, illuminating the practices and perspectives that nurture our well-being over time.

At the heart of sustaining long-term wellness lies the principle of consistency—a commitment to nurturing our physical, mental, emotional, and spiritual health on a daily basis.

Consistency is not about perfection or rigid adherence to a set of rules; rather, it is about cultivating habits and routines that support our well-being in a sustainable way.

One of the foundational pillars of long-term wellness is self-care—a practice that encompasses nurturing our bodies, minds, and spirits with love and compassion. Self-care is not selfish; it is a vital act of self-preservation that allows us to show up fully in our lives and serve others from a place of abundance rather than depletion.

Central to self-care is the practice of setting boundaries—clearly defining our needs, priorities, and limits and communicating them assertively to others. Boundaries are the framework within which we honor and protect our well-being, allowing us to cultivate healthy relationships and environments that support our growth and flourishing.

Another key aspect of sustaining long-term wellness is cultivating resilience—the ability to bounce back from adversity, adapt to change, and thrive in the face of challenges. Resilience is not a trait we are born with; it is a skill that can be developed and strengthened through practices such as mindfulness, self-compassion, and positive reframing.

In addition to consistency, self-care, boundaries, and resilience, sustaining long-term wellness also requires an ongoing commitment to growth and learning. Life is a journey of continuous evolution, and as we grow and change, so too must our wellness practices evolve to meet our evolving needs.

Finally, sustaining long-term wellness is about finding balance—the delicate equilibrium that allows us to honor all aspects of ourselves and our lives without sacrificing our well-being. Balance is not a static state; it is a dynamic process of constant adjustment and realignment, requiring us to listen deeply to our bodies, minds, and spirits and respond with wisdom and compassion.

In the pursuit of sustaining long-term wellness, it's essential to recognize that each individual's journey is unique. What works for one person may not necessarily work for another, and that's perfectly okay. The key is to approach wellness with an open mind and a willingness to explore what resonates most deeply with you.

One aspect often overlooked in sustaining long-term wellness is the importance of community and support. Surrounding ourselves with people who uplift and inspire us can significantly impact our ability to stay on track with our wellness goals. Whether it's joining a local fitness group, participating in a meditation circle, or simply connecting with like-minded individuals online, finding a supportive community can provide encouragement, accountability, and companionship along the journey.

Another vital component of sustaining long-term wellness is the practice of self-reflection. Taking time to pause and reflect on our progress, challenges, and areas for growth allows us to course-correct when needed and stay aligned with our wellness intentions. Journaling, meditation, and quiet contemplation are all valuable tools for cultivating self-awareness and insight.

In addition to self-reflection, it's crucial to remain adaptable and flexible in our approach to wellness. Life is unpredictable, and circumstances may change unexpectedly. By embracing flexibility and resilience, we can navigate life's ups and downs with greater ease and grace, adjusting our wellness practices as needed to accommodate the ebbs and flows of life.

Ultimately, sustaining long-term wellness is not a destination but a lifelong journey—a journey of self-discovery, self-care, and self-transformation. By embracing the principles of consistency, self-care, boundaries, resilience, growth, learning, balance, community, support, self-reflection, adaptability, and flexibility, we nourish the roots of our well-being and cultivate a life of radiant vitality, profound fulfillment, and enduring joy.

As we continue along this journey, may we approach each day with gratitude, curiosity, and an open heart, knowing that with each step we take, we are moving closer to the vibrant, flourishing life we desire and deserve.

Chapter 14

Conclusion - Embracing Holistic Living

As we come to the end of our journey through the realms of holistic wellness, it's essential to reflect on the transformative power of embracing holistic living in our lives. Holistic living is not merely a concept or a set of practices; it is a way of being—a way of engaging with the world and ourselves that honors the interconnectedness of all things and fosters a deep sense of harmony and balance in mind, body, and spirit.

At the heart of holistic living lies the recognition that we are more than just physical beings—we are multidimensional beings comprised of body, mind, and spirit, each aspect intricately connected and interdependent. By nurturing each of these aspects of our being, we can cultivate a profound sense of well-being that permeates every aspect of our lives.

Let's start with the body. Our physical bodies are miraculous vessels that carry us through life's journey, allowing us to experience the world around us in all its richness and beauty. Holistic living involves caring for our bodies with love and respect, nourishing them with wholesome foods, engaging in regular movement and exercise, and prioritizing rest and relaxation. By honoring our bodies in this way, we can support their natural balance and vitality, enabling us to live with greater energy, vitality, and resilience.

Next, let's turn our attention to the mind. Our minds are powerful instruments that shape our perceptions, beliefs, and experiences, influencing every aspect of our lives. Holistic living involves cultivating a positive and empowered mindset, embracing mindfulness and self-awareness practices, and nurturing our mental and emotional well-being. By tending to our minds in this way, we can cultivate greater clarity, resilience, and inner peace, enabling us to navigate life's challenges with grace and equanimity.

Finally, let's explore the realm of the spirit. Our spirits are the essence of who we are—the source of our deepest truths, aspirations, and connections to something greater than ourselves. Holistic living involves nurturing our spiritual selves, cultivating practices that foster a sense of connection, purpose, and meaning in our lives. Whether through prayer, meditation, nature, or creative expression, by nurturing our spirits in this way, we can tap into a profound sense of joy, fulfillment, and wholeness that transcends the material world.

As we embrace holistic living in our lives, we begin to experience a profound transformation—a transformation that ripples outwards, touching every aspect of our existence. We find ourselves living with greater presence, awareness, and intention, savoring the simple pleasures of life and finding beauty and meaning in every moment. We discover a deep sense of interconnectedness with all beings, recognizing that we are part of something much larger than ourselves—a vast and intricate web of life that binds us all together in a tapestry of existence.

In conclusion, embracing holistic living is not just about improving our health or finding relief from symptoms—it is about embracing a way of being that honors the fullness of who we are and fosters a profound sense of harmony and balance in our lives. It is about recognizing the interconnectedness of all things and living in alignment with the rhythms of the natural world. And ultimately, it is about reclaiming our birthright as vibrant, radiant beings, capable of experiencing joy, vitality, and well-being in every moment of our lives. As we continue on our journey, may we walk with courage, curiosity, and compassion, embracing the beauty of holistic living and allowing it to illuminate our path forward.